Love and Learn

Invitation To Super Health

Sergei Komkov-Epshtein

AuthorHouse™
1663 Liberty Drive
Bloomington, IN 47403
www.authorhouse.com
Phone: 1-800-839-8640

Published by AuthorHouse   02/10/2015

ISBN: 978-1-4259-7414-5 (sc)
ISBN: 978-1-4678-1759-2 (e)

LOVE AND LEARN: *INVITATION TO SUPER HEALTH*

PREAMBLE

The book is about love which you should give to your body, and if your body is not yet super healthy, consequently, you have never loved it properly.

We have two duties that should become our missions in the world: a) our personal obligation to ourselves, and b) responsibilities in society that is moral obligations to our extended family that is our local community, country and the world. The first duty is the main theme of the brochure. Both missions are unbreakably connected, internally and externally. In spiritual manner of life it is the same, no difference between inner and exterior sides: a conscience as delicate intimate factor governs public decisions and actions of individuals. Only this type of people will be able to change the course of history in politics and economy and create new human culture.

We live at the terrible apocalyptic time of hatred, terrorism both individual and governmental, wars, mass murders, brutality, slavery (more than 12 known millions all over the world including children). One billion of people live for $1 a day. 15,000 children die every day from hunger and 15,000 more from curable diseases. To finish off this terrible period we need to create new culture of love, starting from our personal relationships with our physical, material essence, and the first step is our health. Weak, ill people cannot produce sound thoughts, feelings and deeds. It is a destiny of spiritual titans who are able to overcome sickness and stay noble and aristocratic. Our general task is to elaborate strong, sound spirit. "Cure yourself first" is the recommendation for everybody, not only for physicians. Thus start from the health and thus prove and prove your ability to manage, rule, solve problems.

The egoistic world leaders, whom we elect for better, are unable to answer contemporary challenges, spending their office terms as comedians. They celebrate the top of their careers, thinking only how to extend it, but it costs too much for the nations. The best illustration of their blind leadership was the last G8. It was a total capitulation before the oldest and most awful, super repressive system in the whole history of the world. The KGB colonel, the best friend and teacher of terrorists, in the role of the President was mocking over the "leaders" of the Free World. All these G7 leading jokers conducted themselves very relaxed without intuition of extra danger. It is not funny, it is very unsafe. The health and life of the planet as a community of individuals in natural environment is in jeopardy. Both human and planetary immune system is seriously damaged.

The loss of normal human instinct of threat is result of the ancient disease – egoism and its derivative – national egoism. We all are guilty, though responsibilities are very different and very individual. Not only violence over human beings endangers the life, but the violence over Nature is already very risky. The mental culture of the Texas cowboy is not enough to guess international crosswords. It is grief of the country (and the world) when cunning is taken for witty. It is time in addition to UN to create the Union of new democratic entities - National and International Communities of Voters who will be able more effectively and decisively to control politicians.

Let us conquer our egocentricity through love to ourselves (!?), to our own body. This is the last chance. We have no other option as to go this way to overcome our instinctive, subconscious selfishness that already exceeds limits of necessary security and thus results in its contrast – surpassing risk. Yes, it requires a conversion of outlook, demands a new vision of mind/body relationships. It sounds newly, but it is already the claim of the modern medicine practice and its recommendations. We must stop to ignore the existence of the smallest components of our living bodies, we have to think and meditate about them, help them and send them wise commands. They are basic actors of our life process.

This brochure is an invitation to join the fellowship of SOUND LIFE (SL) through following EXTREME HEALTH PRINCIPLES AND PRACTICE (EHPP) – SL through EHPP. Every person, nation and all humanity need this change. In the text my personal long experience of healthy life and system is shortly described, proposed and explained as an application and culmination of well known knowledge of some nations. The main aspects of human beings – spiritual, physical/physiological and psychological - are touched. It is known that all aspects should be in the eternal, unbreakable harmony.

This methodology I recommend as the most effective way in education and breeding of human elite.

HEMORRHOID MEDICINE

When a boy and then a young man I was a big reader, the greatest one at least in our family. Being the youngest brother I was a librarian and not only bought and collected books, but kept and saved them. When I detected that my brothers' friends used to take our books and forgot to return I locked bookcase and registered all taken books. Funny to recollect how my elder brothers (the eldest was nine years older) were asking me to give them a book for reading and I registered it in the special copy-book. It was my family's nickname –Librarian. I suffered also when I saw how they bent pages to mark the place of the last reading. I reprimanded them for that and tried to shame and educate.

I read very many fiction both Russian and foreign. Now I don't remember when last time I have read any fiction because the reality and life around is so astonishing that human imagination cannot be compared with it. Finally I regard Tolstoy, Dostoevsky, Chekhov, etc. as the greatest psychologists, and when I open their books I am interested not so much in pleasure as in knowledge about human mentality, and getting knowledge is my greatest pleasure. I am still a big devotee of reading, but my priority is to learn more than to enjoy. With Boris Pasternak "In everything I seek to grasp the fundamentals." After many years of life experience I may repeat after Socrates that when I was a smart young man I was interested in the contemporary sciences such as Physics, Mathematics, Astronomy, Science about the Earth, and so on, but then I realized that the main thing is a human being and all about him/her. Socrates stopped to study these subjects and was trying to understand why it is so that a man knows what is good and does what is bad. I didn't stop totally learning sciences because it is my profession, where I am not the last in the list, but my main interest coincides with Socrates' one and I use to apply my scientific knowledge, methods and skill to investigate human nature and the puzzle. This matter as you see is the same as it was 2,500 years ago at Socrates time (though sciences did really proceed) and the problem will never change its character. Because there is no more enemy for human beings than they themselves, and this challenge can not be altered by any scientific or technological development. The more that too often people use the progress to make terrible things, often creating menaces to the life on the planet in general. The moral ideal of humanity is defined and fixed long ago and theoretically religions are aware of solution, but practically it is a personal question. Now we live in the period of fast, deep and dangerous degradation of human moral and ethics especially among authorities and politicians. If to summon up who were decision makers and had sometimes absolute power in XX century – it is a shame and horror. Some of them were degenerates,

But we were misled not only globally as nations and humanity. Locally, personally we also lost ourselves. It took a long time of our mismanagement over our bodies and deviation from the norm that now the list of human diseases and disorders is so big and continues to grow. There are hundreds and hundreds of different illnesses, and almost every year a new one appears. As a believer I cannot accept that average physical status of the humankind represents God's image. As to Jesus he was physically very strong and endured.

My mammy used to recollect events of my childhood that impressed her most of all. One of them was my request: "Mammy, when the war is over, will you buy me carroty (little carrot)?" It was 1941-42, and I was 3-4 years old. I may imagine how mother's heart was bleeding for her inability to provide her beloved sonny with the simple necessities as a small carrot. Our war generation in the USSR in general suffered from nutrition misbalance profoundly. I recollect my school friends. Almost all of them had big heads and other symptoms of vitamin and protein deficiency. So had I. Thus my start in the race for absolute health was not favorable. I was ill with many of so called "children's diseases", but they are not obligatory at all. About 16 year old I had appendicitis surgery and now I know how to avoid it.

When a student I started to loose hair intensively. For a young man it was a psychological drama. Finally I visited the Beauty Institute in Moscow where I met a true healer among conventional doctors (I strongly believe so) who recommended to get Sn injections and warned that if I would not do that I would loose hair. I failed to realize it and got the predicted result. It is also a very good lesson how small amount of microelements and minerals are important in our biochemical body balance.

When I was about 30 I had a heavy hemorrhoid, and the doctor recommended installing candles into anus. This time I started to read and practice alternative methods and healthy life style. In "Yoga Therapy" I read how to cure hemorrhoid and what is the origin. It was totally opposite approach: not anus, but mouth; not backside, but head and brain should be treated. Thus I understood the narrow-minded methodology of the contemporary Western medicine when symptoms and organs are healed, not the body as one organism. This way "the forest is not seen behind the trees". The Westerners saw details, surfaces of problems instead of looking for roots, first reasons. I chose Yoga and very soon forgot about the hemorrhoid. Now they are recommending colon therapy to list all deposits that result on the walls of our guts. It is again healing through anus instead of mouth. Thousands years ago Yogis explained that poisons and impurities from improper food first go to blood and create different diseases and health problems. The hemorrhoid is the best option because 1) gives very obvious information about dirty blood; 2) as Yogis explained hemorrhoid is the drainage of spoiled blood. Therefore to stop rectal bleeding we should, after Yoga, clean the blood, first, change wrong diet habits that is transform our mind and this way to change the anus situation.

If we will continue to think by backside and try, after official medicine recommendations, to stop bleeding with sticks in anus and then gaily exclaim that we are healthy we will idiotically cheat ourselves and drive the disease in the unseen depth of our organism. Yes, it is good to remove toxic deposits from stomach and digest system, but how? The colon hydrotherapy to clean the colon and the liver, remove debris, toxic wastes and parasites from intestines recommends to apply water cleansing under mechanical pressure. But it is elimination not of a reason, but result, consequences, outcomes. After a while, sooner or later the situation will repeat because the original process of inappropriate stuff accumulation goes as before. Then is pressurized water good? I don't know. It may take hundreds years to investigate what side effects may occur. Again long ago Yogis developed natural exercise "Shunk Prashalana", when drinking water with any additions or distilled one goes through all route without delay as long as you need. Yes, it demands some special technique, but not mechanical, without side effects. There are also other methods of body cleaning as you see below.

When Chernobyl reactor # 4 exploded hundreds Hiroshima bombs into atmosphere I lived in Kiev 100 km from it and was at the peak of my healthy style form. The radiation dose I got is difficult to evaluate, but it was huge. The day it happened I had a rest in the sanatorium near Kiev right on the way to Chernobyl. The road was used by cars from the zone, and radioactive dust in addition to general radiation was brought also. It was a usual crime of the totalitarian regime that the population was not informed at all. What I noticed that new batteries in my radio set discharged quickly and the air became very dry. It happens when air is ionized as a result of radiation. On the first of May 1986 I looked at TV and saw all the highest Communist leaders celebrating the holiday at the open air watching the parade and demonstration. It was the next trickster because all of them took special medicals for protection. My fault was that I still had a portion of trust in them. I didn't know about their preventive measures, decided that there was no big risk and went to play soccer outside. It was the day when winds blew from Chernobyl mainly to Kiev, and radioactive isotopes were delivered massively. When I returned to my job at the Institute of Thermo Physics the special person from the Civil Defense Service was measuring radiation level, but results were never reported to people. Radioactivity meters were unavailable. When I asked him to measure my clothes he checked my jeans and chevron boots, grew pale and demanded to bury boots in the earth. As to jeans he recommended to put them into water for several days. Then he checked them again and finally insisted to repeat boots' procedure. Radiation was everywhere. I continued my running and swimming, but it became dangerous. Than I visited the special doctor who observed me as a marathon runner and "polar bear"/winter swimmer and asked him what to do. He explained that to cease physical exercises is more damageable than getting small portions of radiation. At any case it was impossible to live in Kiev and be totally isolated, and I protected myself by the Healthy Life Style.

THE RULES OF SOUND LIFE

Everything in the world is created by Love, and life is impossible without love. Now a new era has started when we should learn from our organs and even cells how to love. Too long many of Western scientists tried to explain a phenomenon of life mechanically. But all living entities, from cells till humans, have memory, consciousness and will for life.

Every cell of our body loves the body and does her wonderful function because of love, not due to fear or hatred. A cell, which hates her neighbors, is a sick one, may be cancerous. Therefore when I invite everybody to reach extreme, super health it is supposed that all steps will be done with love and for love. On the way of SL you will learn the true meaning of love with your body, which is created to please you and make you happy. But first we should sacrifice our unsound habits and give up false pleasures to provide a chance to our cells, organs and body to function accordingly.

Principles of any doctrine or system start from definition of terms. As to me SL is quiet, joyful and welcoming state of spirit, when the body needs only simple food and sleep. They are the only medications. All regulations that grant healthy life are checked and tested during millenniums. My personal experience is just a confirmation of those verities. In this sense it is my personal discovery and my creative contribution. Nobody and nothing can do it instead of me.

To be successful it is required to apply the FIRST RULE of SL: CAPABILITY TO CONCENTRATE INTEREST. Please, consider how animals, birds, fishes, etc. used to look for food, hunt, do anything in general. They are absorbed with the process wholly, and do not notice what is out of their interest. Without applying this gift it is impossible to reach any result at all.

In SL this attribute should be cultivated and lead to development of the strong will directed to truth. To be healthy we need the iron will to be healthy. The skill of concentration, ability to be attentive and absorbed is a common biological feature, or capacity. Only the deep damage of human nature makes it necessary to mention and formulate.

For a person with a weak willpower and insufficient self-control, it is a helpful idea to find a good company of enthusiasts, a health club, etc. "Keep a good companionship and you will be one of them." Also there are many exercises to train memory and attention, and they may be designed for every specific situation.

The SECOND RULE of SL: LEARN YOURSELF. It begins with the simple observation of yourself, the determination of physical status, endurance, etc. I recommend starting from the simplest deed - a physical health as a first step to develop skill for achievement of spiritual health. It follows from this rule the important, vitally necessary relationship with medicine and physicians. Here I always used to recollect after the great contemporaries and predecessors, saints, scientists, philosophers, poets, etc., that the cosmos around us is a Creation of the Highest Reason, and we are His particles, His cells.

"I am given a body - what to do with it?" Initially this material cover-body, or a vehicle, was designed and created so soundly that it endured for a life-time of biblical proportions. The stubborn struggle of human beings during millenniums against the Creator's Project has led to the sad result of total health deficiency. To find a person with the perfect, absolute health it is necessary to look for as Diogenes with his lantern at the daytime. When he was asked what he was looking for, he answered: "I am looking for a Man". Theoretically all people wish long life, practically we cut short our lives to the least.

Three main components of health: heredity (genetics); way of life; and environment. Genetics has occurred to be more changeable that it has been supposed, and choice of environmental situation is also may depend on us; thus health depends mainly on ourselves.

In the self learning we face the knowledge that we are not body and flesh, but we are spiritual creatures, being given ability to rule our flesh. The deep, very personal and individual experience of this type is known as a "second birth", "birth from above." It is a self discovery, finding of new spiritual reality.

Our bodies are living containers, vehicles of our spirit, and we must keep them sound. Observing ourselves attentively we will know features of our organisms and begin to build our own, personal SL system. Rather than demanding anything from other people, let us learn how to stipulate ourselves. It is about the formation of sound habits instead of unsound instincts that we have inherited in the course of the human history from our predecessors. We need to reevaluate false values first of all. We follow our bad habits because our central brain is enslaved by our local organ's brains and our will is weak. Very often we know what is good and do what is bad. Even if we don't admire the motto "Eat, drink, and be merry, for tomorrow you die" practically we pursue this false philosophy. "Sickness, aches, pains, and physical sufferings are ills that you are responsible for personally. You committed the crimes against your body because you didn't use your God-given reason and intelligence to rule your body with your mind, by living by natural laws." P. Bragg. "Men do not die, they kill themselves." Seneca.

Then the THIRD RULE of SL follows: EVERYTHING WITH PLEASURE, NOTHING ONLY FOR PLEASURE (of flesh). It means that our fleshly pleasures should accompany our reasonable actions as a show of their rightness, but never such material pleasures have to be goals of our activity. Because we are intellect, mental power, spirit, not flesh, then our highest goals and aspirations should differ from animals' ones. Our extreme pleasure should be to think and create, not to digest and consume. This is our head brain that is at our disposal. The rest of our body is governed instinctively well enough by their own local brains. The more that "the idea that the gut has its own brain, or lots of little brains, is not a new idea." Steven Holt, p 176. This is our utmost duty and pleasure as human beings, as top, crown, acme of the evolution: how to send wise command from the central brain to second, peripheral ones. To take the responsibility over our physiological functions like Yogis we should first learn this great ancient science. But to be healthy it is not obligatory to correct our organs brains; let us not interfere in their smart activity. It is according the Highest Design.

The devoted dedication to primitive pleasures is a root of misfortune of many people and whole nations. Those who identify themselves merely, exclusively with their body and fleshy desires, the Indian (and not only) spiritual tradition places into the low class for whom ruling functions in society are prohibited. The violence of this regulation ("cast mixing") for the Indian wisdom is like a national catastrophe. The worst end of world is difficult to imagine. Nobody should allow this sad situation in a personal life as well. It was a tragedy of Russian Empire that happened in 1917; now it is a poor fate of many other nations under dictatorships of low cast representatives. As a result, the health of Russian people now is very bad because "When crows lead the people they bring them to dog's corpse heap".

When somebody lives for the sake of flesh pleasures and other bottom objectives s/he loses sense of measure and self-control, gets caught with different possessions, which lead him/her to uncontrolled loss of energy, inner organs' destruction, physiological and mental turmoil. Such a crazy embezzlement of human being's main capital - health - leads shortly to a personality's bankruptcy.

Our mind should be a conductor of the beautiful orchestra of our body and soul that altogether are created to perform divine symphony of life.

Every extra, only for pleasure, physiological action wears out our organism and therefore the FOURTH RULE of SL follows: BE YOURSELF, DO NOT HURRY, TAKE YOUR TIME IN YOUR OWN RHYTHM. After evaluation of your physical status, or level of health, without haste don't delay beginning of your health recovery. Human's destiny is to manage the body intelligently and to leave the flesh wisely that is in a healthy and calm state of psychic without disturbing anyone around and wasting their time and efforts for care after the powerless body. This is the highest form of an earthen travel final: to go away in a state of beatitude, samadhi.

An age in SL has no significance and is not an excuse for powerlessness and illnesses. "Sickness is a crime – don't be a criminal".

If your consciousness is in a proper state you should be healthy. Never any wise man wanted to return into youth. Youth is a very dangerous period of mistakes and errors when thoughts are weakly controlled, but health is wasted enormously. Store up a health (and reputation) from your youth for in a rape age to enjoy life and enrich it creatively.

EXTREME HEALTH
PRINCIPLES AND PRACTICE

"Our body is a garden where
the gardener is our will."

William Shakespeare

1. A sound mind/spirit

It is not obvious that "A sound mind is in a sound body". First, there is another version that "It is necessary to pray for in a sound body to be a sound spirit". This is a vision of the Medieval Christian monks for a body-mind relationship. Second, this Christian conception coincides with the insight of other spiritual champions - Indian Yogis: flesh is powerful, but spirit is omni powerful. Everything starts from consciousness, and our will is the gardener. According Yoga's model all living beings, including plants and grass, have their own level of consciousness. It is finally recognized by the Western medical researchers that our organs also have their own awareness - the second brains – enteric nervous systems (ENS). Our duty is to properly cooperate with them and live in harmony and agreement. Everybody needs to learn this art of concentrated thinking and meditation over own health, bodies, organs and other aspects of healthy life.

What is "Extreme Health"? It is not so much a state of living without chemistry (drugs) and newly invented medical treatments. The EH is a process of deeper and the deepest restoration of immune system and obtaining higher and the highest level of health. The process is totally individual and personal, though the best way is to make it in groups, clubs, schools, among co-thinkers. At least it should be a family deal. After getting not so much theoretical recommendations, but personal experience and practical skills the student turns into a teacher and may open his/her own Life Extension class or school. Thus your health progress becomes your professional skill with the great privilege and benefit that the longer you live the more precious and important specialist you are. You may start your march to the profession any time anywhere, the sooner the better.

2. Insanity-Doing what you have always done, and expecting things to change

We live in a pretty dangerous, exceedingly polluted environment getting constantly through skin, lungs, and stomach indefinite doses of numerous harmful "supplements" from air, water, food. Often these doses are beyond the sensibility of analytical instruments. Now it is practically impossible to track down sources and ways through which these "supplements" reach and hit our bodies. The list of contaminants in water under the EPA regulation includes microorganisms, disinfectants, disinfection byproducts, inorganic chemicals, organic chemicals, radionuclides. In addition there is a huge list of contaminants which are not subject to any proposed or promulgated national primary drinking water regulation. Totally more than about 250(!) of dangerous poisons. The same with air and food. Autointoxication is the main reason,the root cause of all our health problems and troubles. "Nine man in ten are suicides," - Ben Franklin.

The only our salvation is SL through EHPP.

Among the "supplements" there are exotic poisonous elements that kill the living beings at once plus simply harmful ones that are killing not immediately, but gradually. Thus we should not already expect mercies from the Nature after what was made with It by human beings. Now the Nature needs mercy itself. The scientists and governments in the UN discuss problems of the Global Warming processes. Otherwise the Humankind may get back another great flood to clean the earth and provide a place for a new attempt of the Reason. It goes side by side with catastrophic immunity weakening and obvious powerlessness against cosmic viruses menace for human form of life. Researches are feverishly looking for a way out trying in a desperate attempt to create a sterile, 100% virusless environment on a local level. This is an exit into a blind alley.

"It is better a horrible end than an endless horror"- whales decided and started to throw themselves out of the ocean onto the surface.

Another "joy" is a chemically and genetically changed food for both animals and vegetables. It is difficult to foresee final consequences, but it may be stated for sure that nothing good will result from this new hunt for super profits. Cows following their owners, who get crazy from money desire, have already gone mad too.

Today it is an unconditional obligation, like categorical imperative of E.Kant: before to rule and manage Nature or anything and anybody around, first, learn and govern yourself. The ancient Greek slogan: "Healer, first, heal yourself." The contemporary requirement: "Governor/manager/ruler – first govern/manage/rule yourself".

3. *Natural Health Consultant or Medicine at the Crossroads*

In 2005 I got the Natural Health Consultant Diploma. This is the philosophy that I greet enthusiastically. "Healthcare givers and recipients must have knowledge of all branches of medicine. Currently, modern medicine contains fragmented, eclectic approaches to diagnosis, treatment and prevention. ... **Education in medicine is a key objective for public health.** Knowledge of alternative medical practices and cooperation among the many disciplines of medical treatment can help solve the issues that surround the current status of "medicine at the crossroads." *Natural Ways to Digestive Health* by S. Holt, M.D. ISBN 0-87131967-5.

"To make health twice or ten times better, you need a new kind of knowledge, based on a deeper concept of life. ...state of balanced awareness, more than any kind of physical immunity, creates a higher state of health. ...all of us are responsible for creating the body we live in. …what we build in our bodies we can also unbuild". *Perfect Health. The Complete Mind/Body Guide* by Deepak Chopra, M.D. ISBN 0-517-58421-2

What is an education in SL/EHPP? It is not only theoretical, book education, but also practical knowledge through personal experience under your attentive observation over your own body systems. If you live in family, within family you cannot, but share you knowledge and experience with your beloved. Especially this culture is necessary for children and teenagers to prevent them from mistakes.

"Prevention is a God of medicine". Lead your family members into the country of Sound Life and leave to your children wisdom of super health that is more precious than money and property.

What is the difference between the Sound Life of Extreme Health System and the conventional medical treatment? As practitioner of healthy lifestyle I don't know much about hundreds and hundreds of illnesses, allergies, etc., and prefer to discuss and recommend health technique instead of buying unnatural chemical drugs with side effects. I practice and then recommend the ancient methods of preventive medical and physical culture in the new modern approach.

4. The Miracle of Immune System and our shocking mismanagement

Sometimes I use the term "immune system" in broader sense as ability to resist unfortunate challenges and keep homeostasis, or living force unbroken.

The immune system is a network of cells and organs that collaborate super consciously together as a team, and their duty and goal is to secure the billions of other body's cells, dozens of organs and systems against attacks by external invaders or "guests ", who are tiny organisms such as microbes, bacteria and viruses, as well as parasites and fungi. Those "foreigners" are primitive original forms of life, the very beginning of evolution.

When the immune system goes wrong as a result of both our personal improper life plus mistaken conductance of previous generations plus spoiled environment the smart immune team can not anymore keep under the control the activity of the "foreigners", and it results in a huge amount of different diseases, disorders and syndromes including allergy, arthritis, cancer, AIDS, etc. Now the damage of immune systems has gone so far that Hives destroy just the very immune cells (T-cells). It is an axiom of the healthy life that any inorganic chemical drugs suppress immune systems as well as chemistry including even salt, sugar, etc. in general weakens all cells.

The goal of the brochure is to share the knowledge and experience with everybody, who aspires to be healthy, and show how to repair immune systems and restore the natural order. "Sharing is caring". What is the natural order? It is when a human being - the highest through evolution achievement of Creation - is stronger and smarter than the primitive forms of life, which exists to create an environment for the highest forms. These primitive organisms and cells should serve us, not kill. And when they intrude or we "invite" them by accident inside, our immune systems must be able to resist and stop them, not capitulate shamefully. In his wonderful book "The Bloodstream: River of Life" Isaac Azimov described the phenomenal network that sustains human life, having so many widely diverse duties to perform and perform all of them so well.

Will we help with our central brain to this miraculous system in us to function accordingly?

5. *Life Extension Specialist*

One American paradox: the greatest American physician, the unique Life Extension Specialist Paul Bragg is totally forgotten in his own country, but very well known in the former USSR (Ukraine, Russia, etc). It is because his main book "The Miracle of Fasting" is translated and available almost in every bookshop there. When the members of my fitness club in the USA ask me about my age and system I explain them the origin of my good physical form and other health aspects; then I used to ask if a person knew or heard about Paul Bragg. It is my routine question. I asked dozens of people. All Americans of different age and occupation answers "No". When I ask the same question the people from the former USSR I hear: "Yes, of course." They have his book in Russian language or remember the issue from their living in the USSR.

The famous Russian doctor Suvorin, who emigrated after Bolsheviks caught the power in Russia, was healing all diseases, including syphilis, by fasting. It was the time before antibiotics, and syphilis was incurable.

My dream is to organize sanatorium and realize the Immune System Repair (ISR) course for patients with cancer, AIDS, etc. The success is guaranteed.

If you are not following the Extreme Health Principles or any other complete Sound Life System as a modern implementation of ancient wisdom there is a very big chance that you are proceeding to meet one or some of thousands illnesses the number of which grows and grows every year.

6. Principles and Methods

According the scientific principle to learn the Truth means to surrender someone's egoistic will to the Highest Reason because finally it is not we who possess the truth - it is the Truth that possesses us. "Know the Truth, and the Truth shall make you free." (of errors, also) (John 8:32).

For everyone health restoration is a personal, individual embodiment of the Absolute Truth. It is a duty that should become a mission. There is no age limits; everybody should die that is to exit a physical cover being healthy, quiet and joyful. It is not disappearance; it is a transformation into another reality.

I am 76 in 2014. In the main physical aspects I match 30 - 40 when I was running marathons. To restore my marathon form I need about two months, but it is not my goal at present. According the test determination of the real physiological age I am about 30 in all vital indications. I use glasses to read, but many young people use them also.

My main goal is to be healthy in spirit. In that the most important thing is how you understand and treat an event, which is called "death". "Only who is always ready to die is truly free." "For to die graciously you should die willingly." Christians and Yogis leave their bodies in the blissful states (of Samadhi), willingly and peacefully. It is not a death literally, it is passing away.

In spiritual sense death of the body is a finish of the previous state and a transfer into another reality: we die for to resurrect in a new spiritual body. This transfiguration of our spirit in our earthen body- vehicle happens every morning, every evening and every moment of our spiritual growth that is of renewal; then there is no death, but spiritual actuality that is infinity. For to get such consciousness it is necessary to start Sound Life through Extreme Health practice step by step.

My system differs from new passions-fashions, like aerobics, because there is nothing new taken separately. Everything is tested during millenniums. I only witness that it is healthy and necessary. Only my combination that is a choice of components what is new. The result: more that 35 years of active life without medicaments, physicians, and diseases. Though I used to repair teeth. I have been unable to overcome this inheritance and the consequences of childhood's hard period of thoroughly misbalanced nutrition.

The System includes:

1. A spiritual basis of life as philosophy (wisdom). Everything starts from a thought. Consciousness is primary and basic, and wisdom of all times and nations got together in that. A conscious thought is the beginning of a creative action. "In the beginning was the Word" (Logos, ThoughtSpirit).

Thus the SL starts from the sound thought that is Wisdom. Everybody should always remember that to be healthy is the duty, it must be a dominant thought during an earthen pilgrimage and a start point of self-examination. The SL in the whole is endless creative work, self-learning and self- experiment.

Only we ourselves can create our own Sound Life. Let us start from the first small step: evaluation of physical status or real physiological age. Then we should tell ourselves that everything depends on us, that we are unhealthy because we agree to live this way.

In general there exist three ages: a) chronological (passport's); b) physiological; c) psychological-psychic. The age a) is growing gradually; now statistical limits (life duration) are much lower than biological ones for human beings (about 150 years); the ages b) and c) are changeable; b) changes slower than c); c) depends on emotional state (mood) and may change momentarily. The aim of SL is to lower, rejuvenate b) and c) and their stabilization. In general SL's purpose is not so much duration, but quality, that is the life filled with sense and joy.

Once again: Our health depends on us – this is the philosophy of SL.

Spiritual education is necessary for SL's followers because blind spiritless athletics (bodybuilding) is not sufficient and even comic.

Often it turns into a criminal chronicle. A spiritual understanding of life is necessary for right relationship with own body to say nothing about psychic hygiene.

The contemporary science gives us a unique chance to change our "mechanical" mentality and primitive vision of life. In the course of SL through EHPP we will learn shortly the main principles of physics and mathematics.

What is our spirit? Shortly it is our consciousness + will. Thus we should develop a new mentality, install new "software" product in our "hardware" - biocomputers.

2. Psychic/mental hygiene, control of consciousness, concentration, meditation.

2.1. There are many exercises developing memory, attention, and ability to concentrate and enter into states of a Deep Relaxed Concentration (DRC). These states are translated in English as "meditation", though the Indian Yoga tradition, where it has been practiced and cultivated, has no this term. In Sanskrit Yoga, specifically in Raja Yoga there are terms as Pratjahara, Dharana, Dhiana, Samadhi (PDDS). One of the versions of the meditation technique, proposed to the Westerners, is known as the Transcendental

Meditation (TM), and sometimes the whole culture and tradition is identified with TM, but it is not correct.

Originally phenomenon of DRC is intrinsic to all living beings. It is a biological feature, which again is lost by human beings very often. The scientists and other people of creative professions have these aptitudes as a vital condition of success in their careers.

It is sad that this culture is not cultivated in schools, colleges and universities. In the modern culture they used to spend much time in discussion how to feed our bodies. What about our souls and spirits? A culture of psychic hygiene is still a closed book for the great majority of humankind. The most popular food for human souls is shows, movies, drugs, etc. To admire the Nature around: the sky, trees, seas, rivers, grass etc. we need the ability to focus attention. It also may lead to DRC. This ability is essential in the process of spiritual treasures acquisition; these treasures are given us in abundance. I like fine arts, museums, sculptures, but nothing I can compare with clouds in the sky.

"Poor is this life, if full of care,
We have no time to stand and stare.
No time to stand beneath the boughs
And stare as long as sheep and cows."

It is vital to cultivate skills of DRC, a craft to rule attention and choose priorities to turn them into habits. The simplest exercise is to learn something (beautiful poetry or music!) by heart under self-control. The real prayer in any religious practice is impossible without DRC.

Well, what to pray for? For getting a state of love. Without love we neither can learn nothing nor do something positive. Love is not a relationship; it is the state of soul, mind, and characteristic of consciousness. In brain there are different sites that are activated in separated locations when an individual experiences or love or sexual desire. In another words the feelings of sympathy, compassion, pity and sacrificial devotion are energized with different parts of brain than a selfish desire.

To love means to give, not to get gastronomical and take sexual or other flesh pleasures. Comparatively with the old Greek language the Western languages or even the great majority of world languages are primitive. They use only one term - love, and the same word is used by friends, lovers, parents and children, and fans. The ancient Greeks had four different words for every type of relationships. When Jesus told about love He meant feelings of friendship and parent-child type, "Agape" and "Storge" in ancient Greece. Therefore the first ancient Christians had no confusion about the meaning of the key word and didn't mix it up with "Eros" or "Mania".

If any egocentric person don't use the part of the brain, which is responsible for Love, it gets atrophy and degenerates, may be disappears. It is a biological law that only in-use organs and cells live and develop. Organs out of use decline and disappear. There we may look for what I call 'spiritual genetics'. The modern medical researchers like to investigate different correlations in processes of life. It will be interesting to know how this area of love in brain influences the health and immune system of the person.

The sacrificial love, Agape, brings joy, satisfaction, beatitude. It is very well known that people with this type of character are healthier. This is the folk statistics. "Better to have a circus in the town than to open a pharmacy".

2.2. Thus the capability of DRC is important

for physical health and immune system also. Physical and physiological aspects of Yoga prove it brilliantly. The Western medical knowledge till today cannot explain many of Yoga miracles if in general these phenomena may be interpreted by the language of modern exact sciences. But now the Western medical thought recognize at least the link between mind and body and even develop different methods and techniques to use it (Biofeedback). The PsychoNeuroImmunology (PNI) accepts "altered" states of consciousness and studies the interrelationships among the mind (psycho), the nervous system (neuro), and the immune system (immunology). Dr. Deepak Chopra in his turn legalized Ayurvedic principles and knowledge in the American medical mentality.

The art of the Deep Relaxed Concentration-Meditation develops facility of integral, imaginative comprehension of reality. Then this information is to be interpreted and explained with human conditional languages. All great human discoveries both scientific ones and of arts were done this way. A scientist or inventor accepts image, idea, task solution, discovery as one portion of information and then interpret it into other language. The same is with poet-writer, artist, composer, etc. The difference is only in languages of expression. Every expressive language constitutes a special art and skill. Thus conditional means help to grasp a part of absolute truth and express it particularly. Our abilities to see, hear, feel, etc. are very restricted and help us to act safely in the real every day situation: to move, find food, water, etc. In creative process we go beyond these narrow ranges and comprehend reality wholly, integrally, and imaginably. There is no limit for the process of perfection, and we have to learn to be creators of our own SL. Only through our own transformation we are able to discover the meaning of life and change the world for better.

3. Fasting – time to abstain from food and rest without eating.

Fasting, starvation (in positive sense), time-out, resting from food - this action is also general biological rule for all living beings. In different modifications it is present in all esoteric and practical recommendations of cultures I know.

When 30 years ago I started my SL it was vital to clean all my organs and cells of slag, impurities, poisons, etc., stored in my body during dozens of unconscious life. For this purpose I started 24 hours, 36 hours and 3 days

& nights fasting before I entertained one time two week abstinence from food with watering my digest system. The first week was of dry food abstention that is without drinking. At the end of the first week I started to drink distilled water, then also my urine (urine therapy). After that as a rule weekly I was practicing day and night fasting, three days monthly (later quarterly) and annually one week of rest without food. It took place many years. Fasting itself is the most powerful method of vital force restoration. In addition there are many cleaning methods in other national cultures also. The simple water cleaning during fasting time is quite effective for the beginning though P. Bragg didn't recommend using enema. I think it is up to a practitioner.

All types of fasting are wonderful tools for getting a spirit power and domination over flesh instincts.

4. Vegetarian diet – "Don't kill".

The digest system structure of a human being - the collector of (paradise?) fruits and cereals - is vegetarian. During the long revival process human beings accommodated and turned into all eating creatures. Our closest relatives under evolution -monkeys - begin to eat flesh only when a shortage of bananas and other fruits occurs. As soon as this source is restored they return to plant's food.

Presently nutrition "science" sometimes recognizes the wholeness of vegetarian diet though the multi-million experience of India during millenniums proved it best of all. The Biblical prohibition to eat "flesh and blood" I understand as a ban to use corpses of warm blood beings (which have souls that is emotional and springs of conscious life) was interpreted in Judaism as necessity to delete blood from flesh. Only the Indian tradition keeps this taboo during millenniums.

After animal proteins are swallowed and placed in a digital tract, their decomposition and rotting in long bowels of human beings create there unsound, decayed micro flora which suppress initial vegetarian environment though already spoiled and weakened by previous generations. A bad odor from the mouth is a result of those unsound decomposition processes. In the sound body normally it should be a pleasant aroma from the mouth. Biochemistry of living processes including digestion is so complicated that now there is no the adequate scientific (mathematical) description if it is possible in general.

In everything that relates to living cell, to say nothing about organ and organism, it is reasonable to trust long humankind's experience and apply it individually. Paul Bragg's recommendations about periodical cleaning through fasting are the result of the double experience of all-human and his unique personal.

Natural, not spoiled with heat treatment vegetarian food is the best. I used to eat milk products, egg and fish not every day. To achieve nutrition balance the food should be as various as possible. Supplements also are of great profit.

The principles of natural eating: how to restore it.

When food is natural the taste and olfactory receptors distinguish a product and report human's biocomputer memory (sub-consciousness) all necessary information to keep the balance. If receptors are not spoiled with culinary tricks the information about misbalance goes to consciousness, and we wish to eat something different or special. Now we try to follow "scientific" recommendations, which cannot be complete because of many difficulties. First, there are a great number of still unidentified components of food, and nobody knows when and how they will be discovered. Even if to imagine this fantastic situation when we know everything about food ingredients and their properties and qualities; nevertheless there will be a problem how to apply this knowledge, because every person's biochemistry and tastes are unique.

When diet is balanced the necessary food amount is minimal and small. Hunger is satisfied quickly. It is basic to meet request of hunger, not to play with appetite. "Eat for to live, not live for to eat". When a diet is unbalanced a feeling of hunger doesn't disappear, and overeating starts. The eater stops food consumption not because he/she provided all necessary components, but because the stomach is overfilled. Gluttony may have psychological reason also.

Now it is pretty easy to provide proteins and energy nutrients. It is more difficult to get such unstable components as vitamins and so rare things as microelements (metals, minerals). As it is mentioned before, the science is too far from identification of all food components. From time to time it happens and a new 'panacea' brings next pharmacological boom then often a poor failure follows. It has nothing in common with a real sound life. The scientific knowledge here is useful but it is additional. The main knowledge is our own experimental science about ourselves. 'It is a great wisdom to know myself.' We are given all necessary facilities to discover facts, experience and analyze. <u>This is the 1st step is to restore the role of receptors.</u>

<u>The 2nd step is to be attentive always</u>. Though the knowledge of nutrition facts (calories, ingredients, etc.) is useful, but not sufficient. In natural products there are many unknown ingredients which we may need without knowing its scientific name. Our biocomputer's memory that is central and organ's local brains may give us the necessary advice. The folk experiences of very many nations testify that diverse application of herbs, roots, cereals, etc. gives a positive effect. This 'chemistry' was reliably checked in long history.

In general the common approach to eating when thoughts and efforts are concentrated on getting pleasure should be changed. It is necessary to assuage hunger and thirst, not to please spoiled receptors. A pleasure is only accompanying feature, not the goal itself, indication that food is sound, fresh. A self regulation in products choice and their preparation when your organism hints what to eat and what it needs now is very often violated. In the next issue we will explain what efficiency of stomach functioning is and how many people "run" their physiological systems in vain, misusing food and waste organism. When food is balanced we need a very small amount of it. It should be the first purpose of good, correct nutrition. "The thinner waist, the longer life" – this is the principle of Caucasus longevity.

And a diet may be only individual, personal, exclusive, and unique as every personality is.

5. Frost treatment till winter swimming in an icy hole ("polar bears", "penguins", and "walruses").

The contrast temperature treatment as heat-cold changes gives many positive effects. It is an old (Slavonic) tradition. This is also too big topic, and in this short introduction only contours of therapeutic effects may be defined: 1) massage of inner organs, which is impossible in the traditional manual method; 2) thermoregulation/ adaptation; 3) oxygen balance in blood; 4) sperm genesis - these four are some of healthy effects. It is a very ancient and efficient sport. Like the hardening of iron it creates a special structure of cells or even special cells (protein) itself. It is supposed by Dr. E. Mindell that unique qualities of Himalayan berry Goji are originated from very special temperature conditions high in the mountain when at the daytime it is too hot and in the night too cold. Ordinary plants cannot exist in such conditions. Thus the Goji berry developed special defense molecules which Dr. Mindell named Master molecules.

I personally know examples of miraculous icy water healing when the official medicine occurred helpless. Especially it is effective for digest tract diseases like ulcer. Like in other extreme sports such as marathon running, marathon winter swimming, marathon bicycling; long fasting, etc., a specific biological law starts to act when organism in extreme situation includes reserves, which have been sleeping or suppressed before the physical stress. At the extreme state living beings discover a lot of living power. "If a person wants to live very much the medicine is powerless." In common situations of unsound life these forces are suppressed with harmful habits such as medication overdoses, etc.

I didn't experience swimming winter marathon myself. My observations and contacts with the practitioners prove the great opportunities of the sport though for a 'common sense' it seems incredible. For this type of super extreme it is essential to be a very good swimmer first of all.

6. A heat treatment alone in sauna or steam camera is good itself and matches cold treatment very well. The historical documents testify that "steam camera + a specific type of massage with bunch of brunches ('venik')+winter swimming in icy hole" has been practiced in the Slavonic land before BC. They say that apostle Andrew who was sent to this area saw the procedure. For the beginners it is enough after sauna session to cool in a fresh air.

7. Asanas, static exercises, including upside-down postures. Everybody should trial many different exercises and choose own optimal complex. I did so, giving preference to reversed rejuvenating poses (Shirshasana, etc.). When I practiced half an hour standing on the head my pulse calmed till my minimal rate. It means that the pose is not a physical load. My other preference are asanas developing backbone flexibility. Contrary to the physical exercises there is no tiredness after a static exercises complex.

Especially important is the art of breathing. Everybody should learn "full yoga breathing" inhaling pure air. According traditional Indian literature "prana" is the source of life and energy. Clean air is more important than even food and water.

8. Running and swimming till marathon + physical exercises for key muscles.

Running is a very natural sport, and the marathon sets organism in an extreme situation that awakes its sleeping reserves. It is not obligatory for everybody to run 42 km or more. It may be 20 km, 10 km, but it should be your own limit, personal record. Even walking is good to start. I know examples of miraculous healing (including cancer) with long time running. A choice of lucky combination of static and dynamic exercises is an individual matter of everybody. The simplest of them may be done even in transport. My recommendations are to pay attention to muscles along backbone. They are the key muscles.

Shortly about unique practitioners of Extreme Health who surprised even me - the experienced runner and winter swimmer. It is a winter marathon barefoot on snow in shorts only. Here the brand "Absolute Health" may be fixed. Till today I met only two such brave fellows. Winter marathon swimmers also are worthy of this grade.

9. Sex (prostate) hygiene (ejaculation control + self massage).

The rule sounds as if only for men, but in the deep of the problem it concerns sexual relationships for couples. For men it is more crucial because a prostate named as the second heart of a man became a weak point for very many instead of to be the source of youth and health. Once again the necessary knowledge and experience are known long before. It is obvious that a state of every gland depends on general health level of the whole organism, but at the same time there are special exercises for each. For example, it is known that cold and warm temperature massage (switch of high and low temperatures) is very effective in sperm genesis. Then all excesses are intolerable, and there opens a huge matter of sexual love meaning. Everything is interconnected. "Nothing in life can be abducted; there is a price of everything that should be paid."

There exists a huge area of unknown knowledge for sciences to investigate in future. First, it is a connection between nervous endings of sexual organs and brain. During sexual activity, which is a special type of massage as well, brain cells are also activated plus activity of glands producing hormones. Due to delicacy of the subject the lessons on the matter are supposed to be led in personal communications. I shortly mention that Christian (may be Judaist also) ritual of fasting includes sexual abstinence also.

CONCLUSION

Very shortly: we are composed of cells, and every cell needs 1) nutrition; 2) waste removal. Both processes are made with blood flows therefore active blood circulation and sound blood vessels are vitally necessary. Let us name it as the massage in broad sense. Exercises 6), 7), 8), 9) and partly 3) are specific massage actions that stimulate blood flow activity.

Fruits of Sound Life: when your only "illness" is hunger (not appetite) and your sound food is your drug and medication, which you eat with pleasure, but not for pleasure. Eat to live, not live to eat.

It is not obligatory to practice all sports and exercises. For the beginning one-two is enough, but regularly. Everybody should elaborate his/her own system of individual work-out combination in compliance with everyone's uniqueness. Creation and implementation of individual systems takes the best place among other practitioners as in a big family of co-thinkers.

To change ourselves for better (for worse it goes itself) it is necessary, first, to change mentality and start self-learning and self-training (self-instruction). Our self-feeling cannot be transferred to physicians or anybody else. It is obvious that really we can feel only ourselves. Thus the main thing: start to become conscious and responsibly before ourselves. A doctor may be only helper, consultant, in critical situation - surgeon or re-animator. Decisions and actions with the own body should take on the owner, not hireling. Thus the ancient appeal "To know selves" is the beginning of SL and its continuation because there is no limit for perfection.

To our Ukrainian Association of Movement for Healthy Manner of Life used to come people whom physicians were unable to help. These people caught at us as the drowning man at a straw and found solution-salvation. In a half a year before the doctors who had already buried them in thoughts the fit persons "from the icy hole" were standing and inviting them, sick and sickly healers, to become healthy. Among our activists there were MDs, who demonstrated SL on their own examples and confessed that it were not medicals that provided them health, but the new life style. It took place already after Chernobyl catastrophe, and we extend healthy life of many people starting from ourselves.

Reserves of a living organism are huge. Artificial medicament treatment suppresses an ability to revive, immunity is stifled, and new problems are created. Study, or self-learning, should be combined with the growth of personal achievements in sports described above as well as in other procedures of the SL that will be given in next issues.

It is a consequence of mechanical philosophy that people treat their organs as mechanisms: heart as a pump; stomach as a chemical facility; liver and kidneys as filters; and so on. NO! Stop this vision. They are living beings with brains and feelings. Think and meditate about cells as your partners and about yourself as a spirit that manages your great living Biocomputer – head with brain.

The living body is extremely complicated, open, scientifically (that is mathematically) indescribable biochemical intellectual system, which needs periodical cleaning and repair. Pain or illness is alarm signal, and it should be understood, studied and used for good. But the best of all is to prevent it. You keep your house, car, boat, all your property the best way in the best condition. Why don't you keep your body properly? You spend your time to care after your pets and do it with devotion and love. Give one tenth of your time you spend to keep your property and favorites to your body and it will reward you fantastically. If you are a believer it is your first and direct duty to maintain and honor your wise material substance as a temple of your spirit.

It is only you yourself must restore your vital force because the body is the wise self-cleansing and self-repairing system. With our unhealthy, unnatural habits and preferences we inhibit self-healing power given to all living nature.

One ship pilot was asked by a passenger how long did he work. The pilot answered that was driving ships along this river more that 30 years. "Well, then you should know every sand-bank of the route", - the passenger exclaimed. "No, I know no one sand-bank here" - replied the pilot, - "but I know very well where is the march route".

I've learned through my personal experience where the right route is. Come with questions and knowledge. Altogether we will put down a route of your personal system of SL without or with minimal "sand-banks".

I invite everybody to start a new life through the opening of new relationships with every cell and every organ of your body. They are intelligent and worthy of equivalent treatment. They are doing their best to fulfill their functions perfectly. Present them your friendship.

To love means to give, not to take. Leave behind your unhealthy habits, which lead to physical, mental and spiritual disorders, and give a chance to your cells to function properly. Learn yourself and live in harmony with your wonderful unique body. Your life is a miracle which all sciences are unable to describe.

Through friendly relationships with your cells, organs and body you will learn how living organisms, entities and communities should exist: in love, harmony and mutual understanding. The happy humankind is possible only when we, its cells, will be happy ourselves. The key words: Knowledge then Experience then Experienced Knowledge –K-E-E-K.

After you acquire the skill to look at your body without total identification with it and get an experience as a spiritual creature it will not be difficult to go through what is known as a "second birth" or "birth from above". Here two aspects are important: 1) discovery of new spiritual reality a kind of special mystique experience of meditation; 2) conscious conscience.

We may change the world for better only by our own transformation. There is no other power in the world to change it. Let us make this first step together. It will be sound intelligent international community.

Supplement 1
How to be born from above

The necessity to be born again for spiritual reality understanding was also aired in the conversation of Jesus Christ with Nicodemus who was one of the Jerusalem Jewish community leaders. Perplexity demonstrated in Nicodemus' respond to Christ's words testifies about the decline of spiritual culture, stagnation, which starts always when religious life is substituted with spiritually unfruitful system of bureaucratic rules and trifle regulations - so called 'ritual faith'. In the Indian culture the event of spiritual birth is fixed in the cast system of society: the cast of double-born is the highest, privileged part of the nation. Such a system has already another extreme. When such a totally personal event as a spiritual enlightenment is formed as a cast, estate grouping that is almost juridical, it is too strong extrapolation. Though a spiritual genetics exists, but this phenomenon is more complicated than simple heredity. In India spiritual warriors - yogis - is already above the cast law, and all casts are open to this hero deed. It should be mentioned that tradition to separate and reward spiritual achievements has existed and continues to live in other countries and cultures. In pre-revolutionary Russia it was a noble estate, in modern GB they are knights, though it has no qualification as specifically second birth.

The birth from above completes a creation of human being as an image and likeness of the Creator, who gives sacrificially and creates unselfishly, generously. It is what is mentioned in the Scripture as a specific human Creation. Many animals and birds have soul, mentality and special character. Some of them such as dolphins are so smart and noble that often are more elevated than many people. But only human beings experience the spiritual birth.

Such possession of spiritual life in the depth of consciousness, on instinctive-intuitive level is possible in every religious culture that is focused on the goodness. This phenomenon of enlightenment, edification, illumination, discovery of unseen spiritual reality is connected with a deep innermost experience, which changes life understanding and consciousness orientation. A technological scheme of the process is described in detail in yoga system. Historically Christians created their own meditation culture, and some of them did it independently. It was based on Christ's explanation: "The kingdom of heaven suffers violence, and the violent take it by force" (Matt. 11:12).

Yoga as technically universal system doesn't prefer any religion and doesn't recommend any special cult. The subject of meditations leading to the utmost goal is up to a spiritual activist. It is a mistake when Yoga is regarded as a system without religious faith in an ideal and those who practices yoga doesn't apply for divine power and in his/her spiritual growth relies only on him/herself. It is not true. First, the term "yoga" means unification with the Highest energies and getting beatitude, in Sanskrit "samadhi". Second, yoga is the very ancient science, which experimentally discovered its laws and rules. As an every science it may be applied by different people with different purposes. Christians know that Satan may pretend to be an angel and cite the Scripture. Misunderstanding between some

Christians and Indian spiritual culture, especially Yoga, is due to translation and mentality. When in Indian spiritual texts "Self" is mentioned it is not about egoism, it is about the Absolute that is about God. When somebody opens "Self" inside of His/her consciousness it means that he discovers himself as a spirit, part of eternal Absolute, as a drop of ocean. This philosophy, mentality and practice is closer to Christian way to Jesus than traditional Judaism where a distance between a human and God is never short. Therefore for Judaists the identification with Supreme Being when Christians imitate Christ as the model is impossible. In the ancient Indian source -Upanishad - written long before Jesus' incarnation into a human body there are lines

> The Self reveals Himself
> As the Lord of Love to the one
> Who practices right disciplines.
> -Mundaka Upanishad

The kingdom of heaven (Matt. 11:12) is the kingdom of the Lord of Love (-Mundaka Upanishad). Thus the ancient Indian saints met Jesus in their mystical meditations.

Supplement 2

Dear contemporaries,

both believers in Jesus and not, dear Judaists, Liberals, Buddhist, Atheists, Muslims, and all people who treat their neighbors as yourselves with love and respect and live with them in peace and friendship! I don't want to convert you in Christianity. If you are able to be polite, honest, friendly with everyone in any life situation without any help you are stronger than I am. I have no right to teach you and lead you as a teacher of religion. Because when I am frustrated, scared or angry, I ask for His help. Let it be my personal feature, not obligatory for you to follow it. Let us call those basic ideals which we must follow simply as human principles. I formulate it as a conscience and realize it as God's voice in me. But atheists may explain it as a result of evolution. The more that even among animals we may meet friendship, devotion and mutual help.

Let me share with you my story as with my dear friends.

I was born in Russia in 1938. My father Miron Epshtein was the outstanding industry manager. He was a Jew, non-believer, member of the Communist Party. At the end of his life he started to ponder about eternal life, but I failed to know his deep thoughts. Among his relatives were revolutionaries – Bolsheviks. His uncle Moses Epshtein was the outstanding Bolsheviks leader, prosecuted by Stalin in 1937. My mother was of the Russian noble family. Her father, my grand father, was a Czar Officer. Before 1917 it meant that a whole family belonged to the Orthodox Church. My grandmother of mother's line was involved in revolutionary activity also, and grandparents divorced because of her new vision of family duties. After Stalin's death there was a short period of comparatively liberal treatment of Jews, and I might make a good career in science, army or industry if joined the Communist Party. I graduated from one of the most prestigious technical University in Russia – the Moscow Energy Institute and long time worked as a researcher in Thermo physics. I am an author of about 50 scientific issues and patents. I wrote a thesis and received approval of the Special Scientific Council. According the Western standards it is an equivalent to PhD, even much more. In the USSR every degree had to be approved both scientifically and politically. It was a matter of conscience to represent necessary characteristics and demonstrate my fidelity to the regime. But very early I became a hidden, spiritual dissident, then a Christian dissident. The result was that I stopped the typical Soviet academic march.

My mother, being a hidden dissident, was always critical to the Soviet power, used to ask me: 'Are you, sonny, a believer?' 'Yes, Ma.' 'But those pops...' Here I should explain that this is a very Russian situation, especially for Russian intelligent (educated) people even before revolution. As a rule they didn't respect pops ('pop' is one of Russian name for 'priest'). Actually it was a crisis of official, state Church when believers of all layers of the society used to treat priests with humor, without respect because they often not so much served Christ as made their personal career. My mother also was of not high opinion about pops, but I used to answer her: 'Mom, I believe not in pops, but in Jesus.'

Thus many years I've lived in the "Empire of Evil", which openly counteracted Christ, but at the same time was exploiting the first Christians' idea of Communism. Looking back at the beginning of my way to Christ, I may witness about miraculous, transforming action of the sole name of Jesus. If the heart is open and ready to accept the Word, the Russian art, especially literature, even truncated by atheistic extremists, gives enough spiritual food start a thorough investigation that leads to the conversion of soul.

First conscious seeds of the Good News were sown in me in the Soviet school on the history lesson when 11 years old. It was a short mentioning of Jesus Christ, his death on the cross and resurrection with atheistic explanation that most likely it is a legend. Sub (or super) consciously I didn't take this interpretation and reflected about Him as of a real event. Religious wars, prosecutions and other church's disservices were not connected in my mind with His mission. Those historical costs manifest the damage of human nature.

Under unavailability of the Holy Scripture the Lord's labor is accomplishing another way. I didn't trust the Soviet propaganda and made my own investigation. The crumbs of spiritual truth that remained in Russian and Ukrainian cultures under anti-Christ authorities were sufficient for my spiritual growth. I was a thirsty soul looking for daily bread even in atheistic textbooks taking only Holy Scripture's texts without their commentaries. When a student having read L.Tolstoy's article "God's Kingdom is within us", I used to repeat this title as a discovery, as in the first decades of Christianity when the New Testament was not yet written or available for reading. My university roommates and friends repeated it after me also with enthusiasm without going into theology. Blessed are those who heard and believed.

Jesus came to my life as a result of a long search for the truth in the country of lies. The conscious expression of my faith consisted in the striving for wisdom taken from the origin of origins. Also it was fundamental aspiration to be with and live in the Absolute. Where did I seek under restrictions? Scattered in fragments, God's word might be taken from Skovoroda, Dostoevsky, Tolstoy, Gogol, and others. Though Tolstoy's interpretation of Christ, as I realized later, is not truly Christian and he followed Jesus in his own proud way, without recognizing him as God, but he learned Holy Scripture fundamentally, in native languages, and sited immensely both in his philosophical works and fiction. As we know from the Gospel Jesus was not against when His Good News was proclaimed even this way. (Mark 9:40 'For he who is not against us is on our side'). God's work transcends our limited perceptions, and the Bible gives enough examples of Holy Spirit's actions through sinful people. It is His privilege.

As to Dostoevsky all his creative works in the depth are focused on Jesus. Sometimes Christian literature was available in personal libraries or second-hand bookshops.

At the end of 70th there took place an event, which I call my second birth. It was the getting of such spiritual experience when I met Jesus in the depth of my heart and discovered His incarnation as the central event in humankind's history and, consequently, my personal destiny. At this time I lived in strictly ascetic monk-like way, and I had my first Bible, published abroad in Brussels by the Christian Publishing House "Life with God" and brought in the USSR illegally. I paid for it my monthly salary. The acquaintance with the Turin Shroud Investigation Project, described in the National Geographic in 1978, also helped me decisively. I used the copy of the Lord's image on the Shroud as an object of meditation about events of Golgotha. Tracks of sufferings, tortures and insults over Those Who is the best and purest forced me to suffer. Once during my prayer time under unification with the Lord's image there opened tears in me. A deep blissful feeling of involvement, repentance and compassion in Him overwhelmed me. It was totally unprecedented, both spiritual and physical reading of unfamiliar reality, new

Kingdom, where He is the Lord. This discovery saved me and forced me to see and understand the surroundings and life from eternal point of view. This blissful mode of repentance prolonged about a month. Then this experience and knowledge became a part of my innermost self.

Thus I got the Absolute Source of Grace and ability for transformation of my sinful nature into God's image and likeness. Every time when I forget this Source- the Holy Spirit that Jesus promised to send - I start to feel scare and lost. When I appeal and knock They always give me support, power and wisdom to grow and renew my inner man. This is a miraculous exchange: to give up my own selfish and blind will and instead obtain God's Kingdom.

My personal experience as a researcher-inventor, my investigation of contemporary scientific world-view, and the witness of great scholars has convinced me many times: responsible, persistent search for Absolute Truth, whenever and wherever it has started, inevitably comes to its Corner Stone: Jesus Christ. The influence of His sacrificial love ennobles spiritual frame of humankind, firing hundred millions of hearts.

With Christ we are free even in prison,
without Christ even at liberty as in jail.

Without enlightened faith we are slaves of
sin, prisoners of blind passions. Those who are
deprived of external (civil) liberties are given by
the Lord the blessing of inner, secret freedom.
For Christians a form of government does not
matter: democracy, absolutism, tyranny, etc.
They live in the world, but are not of the world.
But at the same time the deepest roots of the
contemporary Western democracy are in Jesus
teaching and the Christian vision of human
personality. We are brothers and sisters, and
we must treat each other correspondently. We
also are responsible for the Nature around us.
It is God's law.

When open to the Truth that is to the fruits
of the Holy Spirit we enjoy beatitudes: faith and
devotion to the Lord, love to a neighbor, serenity,
inner peace, quietness, joy, compassion, lack of
anxiety and hostility. To win this world doesn't
mean to become a boss or governor, but after
Jesus to be not of the vain world, but a coworker
of Heavens, a performer of the Highest Will. It
is easy to find all these qualities in other ancient
spiritual traditions, such as Indian, and in their
best representatives —saints and mystics. They

do not contradict each other. The Absolute Truth is one for all humankind. The cultural and linguistic differences are not important.

"Don't go outside yourself, return into yourself. The dwelling place of truth is in the inner man. And if you discover your own nature as subject to change, then go beyond that nature. But, remember that, when you thus go it, it is the reasoning soul which you go beyond. Press on, therefore, toward the source from which the light of reason itself is kindled. " Saint Augustine.

Supplement 3

Without Love

1
Without Love we cannot live at all,
Without Love we totally are lost.
Fulfilling duty we result in fall
Becoming irritated in the most.

2
Without Love that charges us with fuel
Responsible person looks like impolite.
And righteousness enhances to be cruel,
Without love it turns in dark that's white.

3
Without Love truth turns you in nitpicker
Who blames and hurts without any aid.

But real truth is not the thing of speaker,
The real truth when blood of love was paid.

4
Without Love we should not be instructed
Because the knowledge will be used in vain:
Not goodness - ugliness will be constructed
And education will result in pain.

5
Without Love the usage of gray matter
Will turn your mind in cunning, crafty head,
But only Love admit to know better
And understand what's good and what is bad.

6
Without Love your smile is not sincere
And may transform the best into the worst.
It is inside that's gentleness of peer.
Without Love all deeds someday will burst.

7
Without Love all competence is funny
And converts expert in a stubborn fool.
One drop may bitter whole bunch of honey,
And only Love is universal tool.

8
Authority without Love is dangerous,
It mars all rulers worse than nothing else.
Without Love all people are never generous,
With greediness that their richness smells.

9

Without Love your dignity is strange,
It is not meek, but pompous and haughty
Or proud, arrogant, etcetera - full range -
To name a whole list of them is naughty.

10

Without Love is questionable faith
And will be put into suspicious list.
You'll never know mercy neither grace -
Without Love you will be terrorist.

11

Without Love we totally are lost.
Without Love we cannot live in grace.
But only Love that gives us Holy Ghost
We feel and know truly hope and faith.
Copyright ©2002 Serge Komkov

Emmanuel or *God with Us*

In depth of centuries this night has gone forever
When tired of enormous mass of hate,
The mass of fury under Devil's fever,
The Earth got rest in Heaven's hugs as a mate.

The many things are now unattainable:
The kings don't look already in the sky
And shepherds in the desert aren't available
To angels' songs about God when fly.

But the eternal born this night of benediction
Is never vulnerable to be destroyed by time.
And word is born again in hearts--it's not a fiction--
Being born in manger long before this rhyme.

The ways of God beyond imagination.
The wisest able to see but only mark
That *God with us* was born for our salvation
And brightest star was lighted up in dark.

Not palace, quiet cave had been provided
To shelter God in tiny childish flesh
For shepherds and for sheeps, which not being guided,
To soften stone hearts and souls to refresh.

Yes, *God with us*, not in remote spaces
Or in the sacred tent with box of trust,
Or stormy breath, or fury fire faces,
Or dreaming memory of centuries that passed.

Yes, *God with us*, this is an open decree.
Among your problems, worries, troubles, and fuss,
You are the owner of the awesome secret:
The evil failed, we'll be forever, *God is with us!*

Copyright ©2002 Serge Komkov

This poem was inspired by the poetry of Vladimir Solovjev (deceased), one of my teachers in faith. By profession I am a researcher in thermo-physics. As Boris Pasternak, "in Everything I seek to grasp the fundamentals." Thus, I look for truth and beauty all my life. Poetry helps me to discover it after Henry Longfellow: Good and beauty are invisibly poured in the world. I used the traditional interpretation that God is with us, though I like more that God is within us and between us. It is within us where main things happen.

Prayer

My Lord, I do belong to you;
Your Kingdom is my only goal.
 I beg, appeal, address to You:
'Give me serenity of soul.

I need it every godly day
To meet all things that in the course.
Please, hear when I meekly pray
And I'll be able to go forth.

When heart is still as it should be
And conscience clean, untainted, and pure
I feel Your presence near me,
I have strong will and I am sure.

When spirit's calm and full of You,
All things are easy to fulfill.
When options, many or a few,
Again I beg you: "Be your will."

Give me submission to your will
And understanding what is measure.
It gives a perfect inner still;
It is my wisdom and my pleasure.

Support my will against satanic,

Without you I'm so weak,
With You I never fill a panic
And will be able to reach my peak.

With You I'm capable to be steady
And meet all news that has to come,
I will be happy and be ready,
With any problem I'll be calm.

I'll meet them with my quiet soul
'Cause it's Your will in everything.
I'll share drinking from Your bowl-
This truly spiritual spring.'

BE WISE with UNSEEN

Please, be wise forever, dear,
It is obvious and clear,
That behind of every scene
There is essence of unseen.

Dear me, or you don't know
That all knowledges of much
Have its origin in flow
From the sources not of touch.

Please, forever be aware
That there is the only meeting,
Only one, divine and fair -
Between hearts in voiceless greeting.

Please, discern two things in mixture,

Make it clear to the end
That eternal is not future
But is within us, my friend.

Supplement 4
THEOLOGY AND SCIENCE:
Psychological Aspects

S. M. Komkov - Epshtein, Kiev
Center of Christian Reconciliation

The report on the 1st Hungarian Conference on Science and Theology, Debrecen., Hungary, 1993, Reformed Theological Academy

> "God has shown you all this, so it is obvious that you have greater wisdom and insight than anyone else.
> Genesis 41:39
> "God's wisdom, however is shown to be true by its results. Matthew 11:19

There is no contradiction between **religion as a way to the God**, and pure or exact sciences, because of the fundamental inability of sciences to solve religious problems, even to formulate them properly. Simply, there are persons who use their education, or illusion of it, to offer excuses for absence of interest in spiritual life and origin of moral and ethics. This is a great challenge for the historical Christianity also.

The aspiration of all nations to live in peace and cooperation has its deepest roots not in political declarations, but in religious conceptions reflecting a mystery of humankind's creation and destination.

The top of secular science wisdom is: I know everything. This frame of mind is vividly expressed by S. Hawking. The top of religious wisdom is quite opposite: I know only that I know nothing (Socrates) that is the sort of negative knowledge. Thus, if I know everything I shall do my own will. When I know nothing I must open my mind, my heart, all my being to the Source of wisdom with prayer: "Be done your will, not mine." There is a special danger of having power by persons inclined to be in the mood of the extravagant "scientific" belief described above. It finally may result in extremism, where extremes meet, including political and religious fanaticism. This is direct way not to the temple, but to the hell, way paved with good intentions. Unlike the expectations of immediate finding of the truth in its final determination, theology sees its way to the perfection as everlasting for ever. This way of theology may be compared with asymptotic approach to the ideal, but the way of a science is like to expanding ball: every scientific achievement enlarges a border of contact with unknown that is the absolute growth of scientific knowledge results in its relative reduction.

Nevertheless, the role of science and its history may be very useful in spiritual life.

They teach: 1) to be insistent, concentrated, and successive; 2) to be cautious in conclusions; 3) to think dialectically; 4) to know the limits of rational thinking. Though these qualities are peculiar in the highest degree to the Saints also, their biographies are known far less on the reason pointed. It is the same reason which led the ancient Greek thinker to say: "If geometrical axioms touched men's interests, they would have been surely refuted by all means".

If we want to estimate rightly the significance of the sciences, including theology, we are to be in the world, but not of the world. It is quite correct in a sense of mathematical logic:

for to prove the verity of a definite logic system we must go beyond the limits of the system. The development of any exact science is similar: when we discover a new law or realize a fresh idea we create new suitable relevant notion & term, that is go out of existing system of knowledge. This state of innocence is an obligatory condition for the discovery of great truth.

There are world's and European's traditions of right attitudes between religion and science. The outstanding scientists, the creators of science, considered these relations first of all, as ethical. In addition, the processes of creative work in both fields of human activity are very much alike, even psycho physiologically, and the author is the same: the Holy Spirit.

Religion and science are not sister and brother or wife and husband. They are Mother and Child who now seems to be lost. But there appears to be a reversal of the direction. The absence of interest to spiritual training and works, being a deficiency of education may be overcame only in mutual understanding and interaction of two ways of creative work: every particular result as in theology as in other sciences, helps to realize the revelation of absolute truth.

Sergei M. Komkov-Epshtein
832 E. Old Willow Rd. # 205
Prospect Heights, IL 60070
USA
Ph/fax 847-229-1519 / 1- 773-791-0244
skomkov@aol.com | www.all-globalconsulting.com

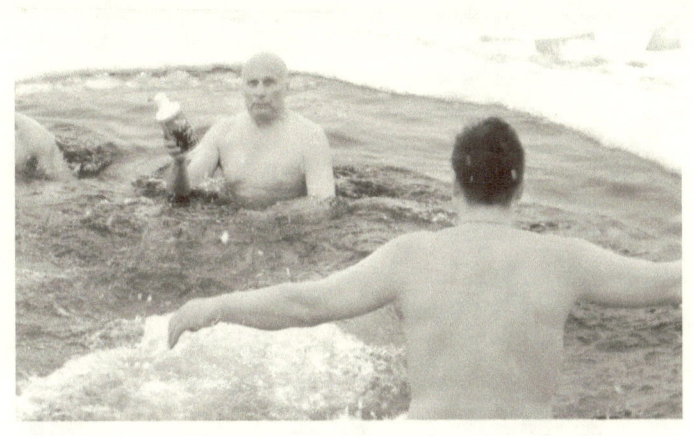

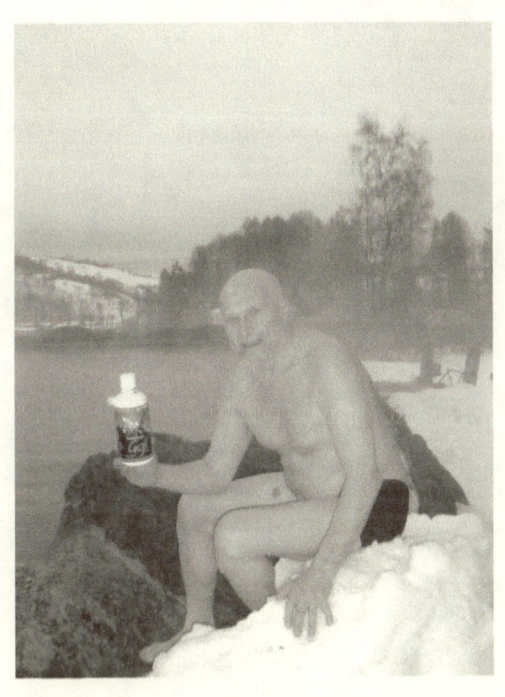

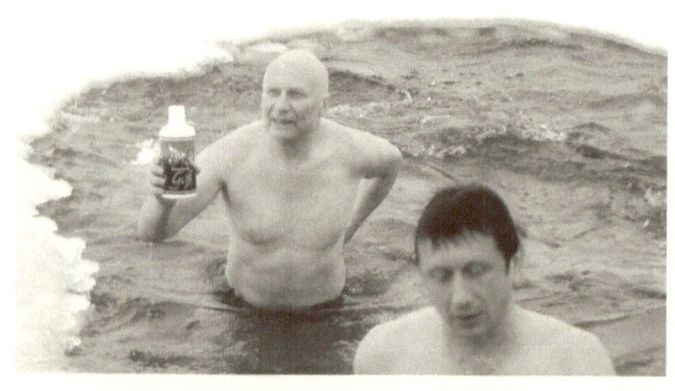

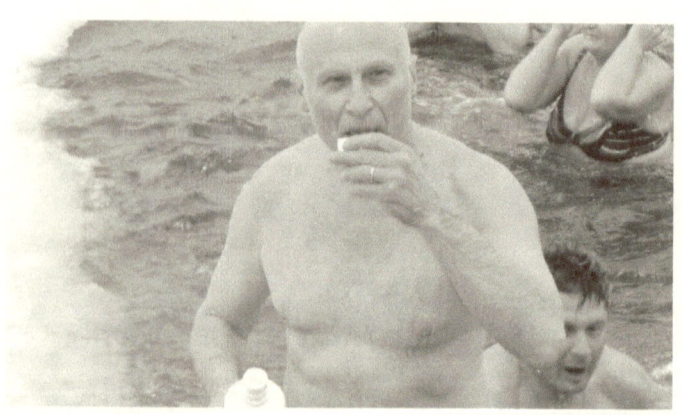

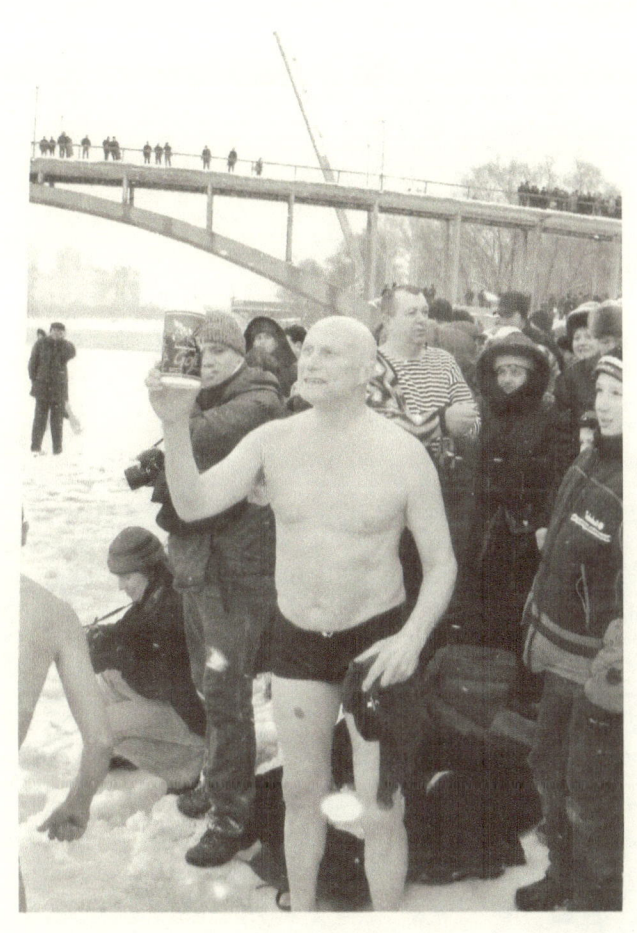

About the Author

The author, PhD in the Power Engineering, all his life looks for the truth: "In everything I seek to grasp the fundamentals". On the ancient inquiry "What is truth?" his answer: "It is a human being him/herself, his/her experience and life (as an initial level of truth). The next level of truth should also contain not details, but the whole entirety of aspects in harmonious coexistence." Truth is a developing process and akin to love is a state of creative consciousness.

Serge made contributions and discoveries in his first profession of scientist & engineer - www.all-Globalconsulting.com .tripod.com. The skill of researcher in exact sciences helps him in all other vocations, including English poetry writing (www.poetry.com, Serge Komkov) and Life Extension line of work. He is also happy having those whom he follows in his spiritual growth. As a result he knows what is necessary to learn and do to become true human best. Many years Serge was running in the Kiev Scientists' House the seminar "Christian Roots of Modern Civilization". His idea how to breed human elite is based on his "know" that is the scientific vision of the history.